10 YEARS YOUNGER - How To Look Younger Naturally [Video Tutorials Included]

Get Rid of Wrinkles With Facial Exercises & Take 10 Years off Your Face in 8 Mins A Day

by Aimee Blake

Copyright © 2017 Aimee Blake All rights reserved.
10 Years Younger

ISBN-13: 978-1976286797
ISBN-10: 1976286794

Look Younger With Yoga Face Exercises, Get Rid of Wrinkles & Take 10 Years off Your Face in 8 Mins A Day

(Health & Beauty Series - Book 3)

While all attempts have been made to verify the information provided in this publication, neither the author, nor the publisher assumes any responsibility for errors, omissions, or contrary interpretations on the subject matter herein. This book is for entertainment purposes only. The views expressed

Table of Contents

Table of Contents   3

Free Gift 7

Introduction   8

Chapter 1: What Causes Wrinkles? 14

Anatomy of the skin   15

Why do wrinkles form?   17

Lifestyle changes to reduce wrinkles 22

A vitamin that your skin loves…   23

Chapter 2: What Are Facial Exercises? 29

Facial massage 31

Acupressure   33

Essential Oils   34

Face Time! 37

Chapter 3: Forehead Wrinkles 39

Facial exercises for worry lines   39

Facial exercises for frown lines   41

Key acupressure points   42

Massage techniques   44

Chapter 4: Eye Wrinkles & Eye Lift 47

Facial exercises for crow's feet   48

Facial exercises for under eye wrinkles   49

Facial exercises for puffiness and bags   50

Key acupressure points   51

Massage techniques   52

Chapter 5: Cheek Enhancement & Filler 55

Facial exercises for cheek sagging   56

Facial exercises for hollow cheeks   57

Key acupressure points   58

Massage techniques   59

Chapter 6: Nasolabial Fold   61

Facial exercises for nasolabial folds 62

Key acupressure points   63

Massage techniques   65

Chapter 7: Laugh Lines & Lip Fillers 67

Facial exercises for laugh lines and lipstick lines   68

Key acupressure points   70

Massage techniques   71

Chapter 8: Define Jaw & Double Chin 73

Facial exercise for jaw definition 74

Facial exercises for double chin   76

Key acupressure points   77

Massage techniques   78

Chapter 9: Tighten Neck Skin 80

Exercises for crepey, wrinkling neck skin   81

Exercises for turkey neck   82

Key acupressure points   83

Massage techniques   85

Chapter 10: Step-by-step 8 Minute Routine   87

8 Minute Routine Break Down By Minute   89

Other Books By Aimee   101

Free Gift   103

About The Author   104

Free Gift

Get the "8 Point Facial Acupressure Routine" for Free at:
http://bit.ly/8ptacupressure

- The facial acupressure routine are for the days you don't want to perform facial exercises.
- The best part it only takes 2 minutes to complete!

Download it for free now at:
http://bit.ly/8ptacupressure

Introduction

Although wrinkles is a part of the natural aging process, it *doesn't* mean you can't do something about it. There **IS** a way to age gracefully and look 10 years younger than your biological age.

At the time of writing August 2017, I'm 35.5 years old 😌 and have been told by people who meet me for the first time that I look 25.

I've pulled out photos from my mid twenties to compare it with photos of how I look like now so that you can be the judge of it.

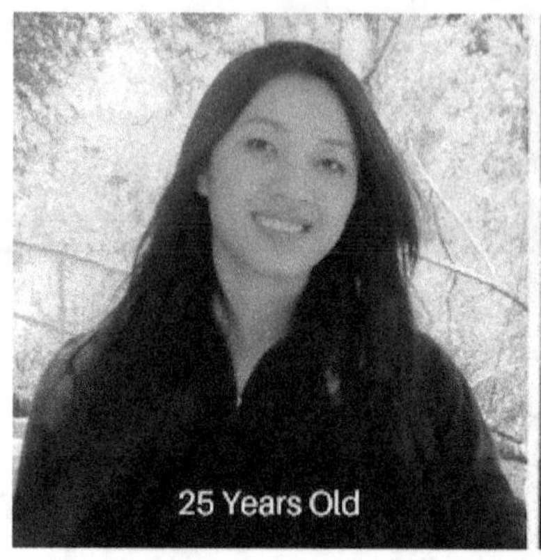
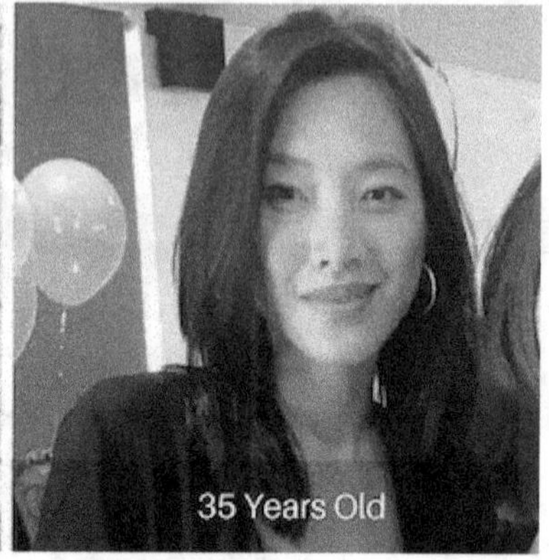

No fillers, botox or any photo editing. These are my original photos.

In my early twenties, my diet wasn't healthy. I ate a lot of junk, smoked cigarettes and drank alcohol and took my face and body for granted.

By the time I turned 30, I was 20 pounds heavier, my acne had worsened and lines began to form around my mouth and underneath my eyes.

Preventing wrinkles and premature aging is simple if you know how. You need 2 things: a clean healthy diet and facial exercises.

You can find my diet on Amazon kindle by searching for "Vogue Hack - Lose 10 pounds in 10 days Aimee Blake". However for the purposes of this book, I will be focusing on how you can look 10 years younger using facial exercises.

Perhaps it's the big skin care companies brain washing us but women are led to believe that their facial skin is extremely delicate and can only touched gently by a beauty therapist or professional.

We don't trust our own hands near our face and wouldn't dream of holding firmly on our skin or exercising our facial muscles. But the secret of looking 10 years younger lies within you not some expensive toxin laden cream.

We place our facial skin in a separate category, we believe that it is super delicate and not living at all which is far from the truth.

Your facial skin is an organ of the body and requires maintenance as well. Just like the rest of your body, your facial skin is attached to tiny facial muscles by connective tissue.

It behaves like other organs of the body, heart, lungs and skeletal muscles and maintain it's firmness, suppleness and

skin elasticity through stimulation and
exercise.

Getting older doesn't mean you have to
put up with wrinkles or resort to
spending a fortune on creams, devices
or cosmetic treatments to look 10 years
younger.

When you exercise your face, you
strengthen the relationship between the
skin and muscles in unison, improving
tone and increasing circulation.

The purpose of this book is to show you
how facial exercises can transform your
facial contours, get rid of wrinkles and
help you achieve a more vibrant
complexion though simple and easy to
follow steps.

However I like to stress that consistency is the key, these exercises may seem simple but the cumulative effect of all these exercises combined will give you a non surgical face lift without the down time so please be patient.

Are you ready? Lets begin!

Chapter 1: What Causes Wrinkles?

No one likes the idea of getting older, and we certainly don't want our faces to look older than our actual age.

However, few of us relish the idea of botox shots, filler injections, and surgical facelifts either. Don't worry – this book shows you a free, natural and non-invasive alternative to anti-aging.

But before you can attempt to prevent and reduce wrinkles, it is important to take a closer look at what causes them. In this chapter, you will learn about:

- the anatomy of the skin

- the factors which contribute to wrinkles and
- Some natural at-home remedies for boosting a healthy, youthful complexion.

Anatomy of the skin

The skin is responsible for multiple functions within the body. These include perception of touch and sensation, temperature maintenance, regulation of the body's salt-water balance, and protection from infection.

The skin is comprised of a number of layers, namely the epidermis, dermis, and subcutaneous tissue, as well as other structures such as hair follicles, sweat glands, and pores.

The skin also contains sebaceous glands, which produce the natural oils that hydrate your skin. Sebaceous gland activity is what contributes to the various skin types – normal, combination, dry, and oily.

The epidermis is the outermost layer of the skin and is therefore at highest risk of wear and tear. It is essentially a barrier between the body and the outside world. This is also the layer with the highest rate of cell removal and renewal.

Underneath the epidermis lies the dermis. The dermis is principally involved in perception, defense, and thermoregulation.

The structure of the dermis includes bundles of collagen proteins interspersed with elastin fibers. These give the skin its firmness and elasticity.

Finally, the subcutaneous tissue is a fatty layer below the dermis. This layer stores lipids, and protects and insulates the body.

Why do wrinkles form?

Wrinkling occurs when skin loses its elasticity and resilience. Temporary lines can be seen whenever we contract our facial muscles by forming an expression.

Over time, the mechanical stress of repeated muscle contraction causes these expression lines to become visible at rest, forming a permanent wrinkle.

This process is affected by both the physiological functions of the body (intrinsic factors) and the skin's exposure to the environment (extrinsic factors). These intrinsic and extrinsic factors interact and work simultaneously, affecting the rate and mechanism by which wrinkles form.

Many of the natural processes of aging are the primary contributors to wrinkle formation.

At an epidermal level, the rate of cell renewal and sebaceous gland activity slows, resulting in looser, drier skin. This is augmented by weakened attachment between the dermis and epidermis.

The skin is therefore more vulnerable to damage, deformation, and poor healing. Studies have also shown that dry, fair, alkaline skin has a greater rate of wrinkle formation than other skin types.

In the dermis, there is a reduction in collagen and elastin production. Younger skin has well organized, dense collagen structures.

As we age, these collagen bundles become thinner and less coordinated, and the elastin fibers lose their ability to return to their original state.

There is also a loss of superficial fat to the face due to reduced blood flow, hormonal changes, and lowered metabolism, which results in hollowness in the cheeks and more visible lines.

Although it would be incorrect to say that extrinsic factors such as sun exposure and smoking are the cause of wrinkles, it cannot be denied that they greatly accelerate the process.

Smoking damages the blood vessels which oxygenate the skin, and decreases collagen and elastin production.

So regular smoking can speed up the aging process by ten to fifteen years *(In my earlier years I had a horrible habit of chain smoking)*

On top of this, smoking greatly increases your risk of developing other skin disorders, such as psoriasis, viral infections, and skin cancers. If you haven't quit, now would be a good time to.

UV damage, or photo-aging, is responsible for changes in the skin's molecular integrity. This reduces the cells' ability to accommodate stress and hold water, and leads to the synthesis of dysfunctional elastin proteins.

As well as aggravating the intrinsic causes of wrinkle formation, photo-aging also results in dry rough skin, deeper wrinkles, irregular pigmentation, and a higher risk of malignant growths.

Lifestyle changes to reduce wrinkles

No targeted wrinkle-reducing exercises will have a long lasting effect if your health and environment are not addressed. As explained above, cigarettes and UV light do detrimental damage to your skin.

Kick the smoking habit, stop the sun beds, and smother yourself in SPF if you really want to reduce wrinkles and gain a glowing youthful visage.

Vitamins can have a hugely positive impact on the condition of your skin. Antioxidants such as Vitamin A have been shown to reduce fine wrinkle and dark circles under the eyes.

Vitamin C and Vitamin E, also antioxidants, have the ability to reduce UV damage by destroying harmful free radicals, preventing further collagen and elastin breakdown.

There is also evidence to suggest that when used in combination, Vitamin C and E can reduce the risk of basal cell carcinoma.

Vitamin B3 (also known as niacin) enhances the skin's ability to store moisture, lowering the risk of skin breakdown and reducing dryness.

A vitamin that your skin loves...

In my "Radiant Skin - Acne Treatment Book by Aimee Blake", I discovered a break through for beating acne using Niacin (B3).

Well niacinamide, also known as vitamin B3 plays an important role in cellular energy production.

It has anti-inflammatory properties, which makes it effective for not only treating acne but it had a skin tightening and firming effect on mature skin.

This is one of my hidden secrets used in conjunction with the 8 min daily facial exercises routine.

After performing facial exercises, I would apply a natural home made a

Niacinamide serum at 5% to assist in cell renewal.

* **Personal tip:** I make my own Niacinimide serum at 5% strength - all of the ingredients can be purchased online via amazon or iherb.

The below recipe is simple and has kept my skin baby smooth and blemish free. Niacinimide powder comes in a fine white powder and dissolves easily in distilled water.

Recipe: Niacinimide Serum 5%
You will need a scale. Ingredients:
- 5% Niacinimide powder
- 2% Hyaluronic acid
- 93% Distilled Water

Instructions:

- Mix everything together until dissolved
- Store in a sterilized jar and refrigerate.
- Should keep up to 2 weeks.
- Apply the serum on a clean face at night before bed

Niacinimide Products

If you don't have a sterile environment and prefer to buy your own niacinimide serum, I recommend these 2 products:

1. Acnessential 4% Topical Niacinamide cream
2. Skin Daily Niacinamide Vitamin B3 Cream Serum 5%

I spent some time researching the best niacinimide serums and these two are the best on Amazon - they have high quality ingredients, positive reviews and are affordable.

Other vitamins can be taken orally or used in a lotion and rubbed directly into the skin. Make sure to adhere to recommended daily allowances.

Stress reduction is also an important factor in the fight against aging skin. High levels of stress can increase inflammation and exacerbate any existing problems. Practice slow, intentional breathing, meditation, or yoga to reduce anxiety and worry, and keep your face and body in top shape.

Finally, don't skimp on your beauty regime. A good pH Balanced moisturizer counteracts the drying effect of aging and prevents cracks and cuts forming.

Before undertaking your short facial exercise routine (which we'll discuss in the next chapter), keep your skin happy by cleansing, toning, and moisturizing your face and neck every day.

Chapter 2: What Are Facial Exercises?

Facial exercises are a series of movements designed to increase circulation, improve complexion, and give you a surgery-free facelift.

The first published record of facial exercises is from a French pamphlet in 1710, although some claim that the practice dates all the way back to Cleopatra.

These regimes have been developed and innovated ever since, and there is now a plethora of programs available.

Facial workouts are based on the
principle that the muscles of the face
can be trained not to fall into the
patterns that create lines and wrinkles.

An increase of blood and oxygen to the
face and neck also tones the skin and
nourishes the cells to create that
youthful glow.

Dermatologists and estheticians
worldwide have long known the benefit
of facial exercises and are now offering
treatments and courses in facial yoga
and natural facelifts (combined with
cosmetic serums).

To enhance the effectiveness of these
exercises, I also discuss the benefits of
facial massage, acupressure, and

aromatherapy in the reduction of wrinkles.

In the following chapters, you will learn an easy, at-home routine to reduce your wrinkles, firm your neck, and altogether rejuvenate your skin – all in eight minutes!

Facial massage

Some of the reasons to integrate facial massage into your daily routine include reducing puffiness, improving circulation, and tightening skin.

In addition to the aesthetic benefits, massage has also been proven to stimulate sebaceous gland production, lower stress levels, and reduce muscular tension.

Why does rubbing your face work?
By stimulating specific lymph nodes,
toxins and excess fluid are drained
away, diminishing swelling and
puffiness.

Massage also improves blood flow to
the area, increasing oxygenation to the
cells, which in turn promotes healing
and brightens a dull complexion.

Like any type of massage, there are
many traditions and styles associated
with facial massage, each with their own
techniques and benefits.

These can vary from the long, soothing
strokes of Swedish massage to the

pressure point stimulation of Japanese Shiatsu.

In the following chapters, we lay out the most effective combination of these techniques for each area of your face, so you can get the most out of your facial workout.

Acupressure

Rooted in traditional Chinese medicine, acupressure is based on the concept of energy pathways, or meridians, which flow through the body.

By stimulating specific points along these meridians, we can clear any blockages and restore balance to the body. Other practices, such as Shiatsu massage and reflexology, are based on similar theories.

Although Western medicine has mixed views of acupuncture and acupressure, studies have shown the practice's effectiveness in stimulating endorphin release, and consequently reducing pain and nausea.

While facial exercises and massage primarily vitalize muscles, acupressure is the perfect supplement to activate lymphatic drainage and boost the nervous system, creating a complementary combination to curtail wrinkles.

Essential Oils

Essential oils help promote relaxation, reduce depression, and, of course, treat skin conditions.

As well as being useful treatments for psoriasis, scarring, and inflammation, a variety of essential oils can be used in wrinkle reduction.

Although a thorough explanation of the uses of aromatherapy is beyond the scope of this book, the following three essential oils are the perfect thing to take your daily facial routine to the next level.

Rosehip seed oil:
High in omegas 3 and 6, and loaded with Vitamins A and C, rosehip seed oil is noted for its ability to reduce the

appearance of scars, sun damage, and wrinkles. It is also a fantastic moisturizer for dry and/or mature skin.

Patchouli oil:

This antiseptic, diuretic essential oil has been shown to promote healing, break down cellulite, and hydrate dry and cracked skin, and is particularly useful in the treatment of dermatitis, eczema, and acne scars. It also stimulates skin cell renewal, a process that slows with age.

Neroli oil:

This sweet, soothing oil increases circulation, promotes smooth skin, and reduces the appearance of broken capillaries, stretch marks, and scars. It is effective as an emollient, cleanser, and toner.

All of the above methods can be carried out on dry skin, with light oils, or while moisturizing, but if you do want to explore the benefits of aromatherapy, remember to dilute your essential oils in carrier oils (such as jojoba oil or sweet almond oil) or in a lotion, so as to avoid unpleasant skin reactions.

Face Time!

So, what is your eight-minute facial routine going to involve? In the following chapters, you're going to learn:

- Acupressure points
- Massage techniques
- Reducing forehead wrinkles
- Lifting the eyes
- Exercises to enhance and plump up cheeks

• Exercises to diminish a double chin

• And exercises to tighten the neck

As you progress, there will be a lot of overlap in the function of the muscles and ligaments of the face. This means that aging in one area will likely impact on another area.

Therefore, in the final chapter, you're going to get the step-by-step 8 minute routine which summarizes the main exercises to looking 10 years younger.

Chapter 3: Forehead Wrinkles

Forehead wrinkles can be categorized into two main types:

- transverse "worry" lines which lie perpendicular to the frontalis muscle
- and oblique "frown" lines which lie perpendicular to the corrugator muscle.

Each exercise is designed to train your muscles into remaining smooth rather than falling into the expressions which cause wrinkles over time.

Facial exercises for worry lines

- In front of a mirror, wide your eyes as much as possible without wrinkling your forehead.
- To work on this exercise, place your thumb on your brow and index fingers on the outer edges of your forehead near the hair line to keep it steady.
- Using light pressure, start contracting your forehead as you raise your eyebrows up and down.
- During this process, be mindful of not wrinkling your forehead whilst performing this exercise.
- Hold for five seconds before releasing.
- Repeat the above exercise three times.

- To perform this facial exercise, please watch the video tutorial at: **http://bit.ly/worrylines**

Facial exercises for frown lines

- First Part: In front of a mirror, place your your index and middle finger firmly down in your frown area
- Then attempt to frown and be mindful of not wrinkling your forehead any further.
- Hold for five seconds before releasing.
- Repeat the above exercise three times.
- Second Part: Pinch the innermost corners of your brows with your index and middle fingers.

- Start contracting your frown area whilst pulling them away from each other
- Hold for ten seconds before releasing.
- Smile! Think happy thoughts and smile as wide as you can, smoothing out the forehead.
- Repeat the above exercise three times.
- Bonus tip: Incorporate this into your day – your forehead can't wrinkle if your smiling and you'll gain a reputation for being bright and friendly.
- To perform this facial exercise, please watch the video tutorial at: **http://bit.ly/frownline**

Key acupressure points

The first point that we can use to reduce lines in the forehead is the Yin Tang point. This pressure point is located directly between the eyebrows, and is connected to the pineal nerve which stimulates melatonin production.

- Melatonin (available in capsules and liquid form) is the hormone involved in sleep regulation and aids in stress reduction. It is antagonistic to cortisol, a hormone that responds to stress and is involved in the "fight or flight" reaction of the body.
- Using your index fingers or thumb, put pressure on the spot between your brows.
- The pressure should be firm, but not overtly painful.

- Make ten small circles on the spot
  before releasing.
- Bonus tip: taking melatonin liquid
  helps regulate your sleep and has
  anti-acing benefits.

The second pressure point is called
Taiyang and is located at the temples.
Stimulating this point will help reduce
stress and tension, as well as boosting
circulation and concentration.

- Use your index and middle fingers to
  make ten small circles at each temple
  before releasing.

Massage techniques

Using a pH Balanced moisturizer or light
oil like Rosehip seed oil will allow your
hands to glide more easily over your

face, but these maneuvers can be
carried out on dry skin.

- Using the pads of your fingers, make light circular strokes from the center of your forehead out towards your temples.
- Move outward and upward to lift the face.
- Using the same technique, start at the bridge of your nose and massage up and out to your hairline.
- Placing your index, middle, and ring fingers at the point of your frown lines, apply light pressure and pull your fingers out towards your temples.
- Again using your three fingers, lightly pat the skin of your forehead to rejuvenate the skin.

- Using your index and middle fingers, lightly pinch along the length of your eyebrows.
- Use enough pressure to create friction on the muscle but avoid going so hard that you would cause pain or bruising. Continue along the length of your hairline.

Chapter 4: Eye Wrinkles & Eye Lift

Eyes are the window to the soul, and are also a big giveaway when it comes to our age. The skin around the eyes is some of the most sensitive and delicate skin in the body, making it one of the first spots to develop wrinkles.

This chapter will address the three main signs of aging around the eyes.

"Crow's feet" are the lateral lines that lie perpendicular to the orbicularis oculi muscle. Wrinkles associated with the same muscle can also form under the eyes.

Puffiness or "bags" under the eyes can occur for a number of reasons, including tiredness and water retention.

As we age, bags are often caused by loosening in the ligaments and muscles of the face which make fat deposits under the eyes more visible.

The following exercises are designed to combat these signs of aging by strengthening the muscles around the eyes and discouraging fluid retention.

Facial exercises for crow's feet

- In front of a mirror, place your thumbs or index fingers on the outer edges of each eye
- Hold down the skin down firmly with your fingers

- Then close your eyes tightly whilst holding the corners of your eyes down firmly to prevent wrinkling
- Hold skin for five seconds before releasing
- Then repeat three times.
- To perform this facial exercise, please watch the video tutorial at: **http://bit.ly/crowfeet**

Facial exercises for under eye wrinkles

- With your eyes closed, raise your eyebrows up while stretching your eyelids downwards.
- Hold for five seconds before releasing.
- Place an index finger at the outer corner of each eye.

- Lightly pull your fingers up as you press your eyelids shut.
- Hold for five seconds before releasing.
- To perform this facial exercise, please watch the video tutorial at: **http://bit.ly/undereyewrinkles**

Facial exercises for puffiness and bags

- Facing straight ahead, open your mouth in a wide 'O' shape.
- Then tilt your head slightly back and eyes looking up
- Hold for five seconds before releasing
- Repeat the above exercise three times.

- To perform this facial exercise, please watch the video tutorial at: **http://bit.ly/puffeyebags**

Key acupressure points

The first acupressure point comes from the Japanese tradition of Shiatsu. The "Shi-Haku" point lies below the socket, at the center of the eye. It is also known as Sibai in Chinese Traditional Medicine.

Stimulating this point will help to reduce dark circles under the eyes, and other facial blemishes such as acne. Use your thumb or middle finger to apply firm pressure to the area and make ten small circles under each eye before releasing.

The second pressure point, Jing Ming, is located at the bridge of the nose, at the inner corner of the eye. Activating this point will relieve tense and tired eyes, and eliminate crow's feet.

Place firm pressure on either side of the bridge of the nose using your index fingers. Make ten small circles before releasing.

Massage techniques

Use a lighter touch around the eyes to protect sensitive skin. If you choose to you use a pH Balanced moisturizer or light oil like Rosehip seed oil, be careful to avoid getting any substances in the eyes.

- Using your middle fingers, make very light circular movements around the eye.
- Move upward and outward to lift the face.
- Start at the outside edge, moving under the eye to the tear duct.
- Work your way up the bridge of the nose towards the outside edge of the eyebrow.
- In the same direction, use the pads of your index fingers to lightly tap around the eyes.
- Start at the outside edge of the eye and work your way around as above.
- To drain fluid, use your middle fingers to apply small amounts of pressure to the bones of the eye socket.
- Start at the inside of the eye, press, lift your fingertips and move to the

next spot, working your way out the edge of the eye.

• Repeat this movement, starting at the bridge of the nose and working your way down towards the nostrils in order to clear the sinuses.

• Rub your hands together to build up heat. Place your palms over your eyes to allow them to absorb the warmth. Make sure you do this with dry hands.

Chapter 5: Cheek Enhancement & Filler

Cheeks may not wrinkle as much as other parts of the face, but we can see dramatic changes in the shape of the face as we age. Two processes may occur.

The first is the sagging of the cheeks. This is due to increased laxity in the muscles and ligaments of the face combined with the effects of gravity.

These ligaments are some of the weakest in the face and are particularly susceptible to drooping, leading to the formation of jowls.

Secondly, there can be noticeable hollowing of the cheeks. This hollowness is created by fat loss under the subcutaneous tissue, and decreased collagen and elastin synthesis.

The following exercises aim to brighten the skin and strengthen the muscles of the face to keep your complexion looking youthful and vibrant.

Facial exercises for cheek sagging

- First Part: Open your mouth as wide as possible. Stick out your tongue and look upwards.
- Hold for ten seconds before releasing.
- Bring your bottom lip over your top lip and smile as wide as possible.

- Hold for five seconds before releasing.
- Second Part: Pinch the fleshy parts of the cheek under the cheekbones with your thumb and index finger. As you pull the skin outwards and try to tense your cheeks up.
- Hold for five seconds before releasing.
- To perform this facial exercise, please watch the video tutorial at: **http://bit.ly/cheeksag1 + http://bit.ly/cheeksag2**

Facial exercises for hollow cheeks

- Puff your cheeks out as far as you can. Move the air to cheek and hold ten seconds before releasing.

- Then holding the side of your cheeks, your mouth forming and O and tensing up and down for 5 seconds.
- Use your lips to cover your upper and lower teeth. Smile as wide as you can and hold for ten seconds before releasing.
- To perform this facial exercise, please watch the video tutorial at: **http://bit.ly/hollowcheeks**

Key acupressure points

The first acupressure point for the cheeks is Ju Liao. Nicknamed "Facial Beauty", this point is located below the pupil and in line with the nostril, in a slight depression.

Stimulation of this point increases circulation, and reduces swelling and congestion of the face and sinuses.

Using your thumb or middle finger, apply firm pressure to the area. Make ten small circles before releasing.

Massage techniques

Using a pH Balanced moisturizer or light oil like Rosehip seed oil will allow your hands to glide more easily over your face and cheeks, but these maneuvers can be carried out on dry skin.

- Using firm upward strokes, massage from your jaw up to your cheekbones using small circular motions. Cover the entire area of the cheek using upward, outward motions.

- Place your index, middle, and ring fingers at nostril level at either side of the nose. Slowly and firmly, pull your fingers across the cheekbones, out towards the temples.
- Invigorate and detoxify the skin by tapping along the cheeks with the pads of the fingers. Work your way back and forth along the cheekbones before covering the whole cheek.
- Lightly pinch along the cheeks to encourage circulation and color.
- Very gently, knead the cheeks with your knuckles. Do not go so deeply that it is painful.
- Finish with long strokes with the palms of your hands to relax the face.

Chapter 6: Nasolabial Fold

The nasolabial fold is the area connecting the corner of the lips to the edge of the nostrils. Nasolabial lines lie perpendicular to the zygomaticus muscle.

Although people of all ages have these lines, as we get older, the nasolabial folds can become more pronounced.

After a period, they can even extend far enough down the chin to form "marionette" lines or jowls (which we will tackle in the next chapter).

Another reason for the development of nasolabial lines is sagging of the cheeks (see chapter 5) which adds heaviness and weight to the face.

The following exercises aim to strengthen the muscles and smooth the skin to prevent unwanted deepening of these wrinkles.

Facial exercises for nasolabial folds

- Purse your lips as if you were going to blow a kiss. Looking straight ahead, move your lips up, like you are trying to kiss the ceiling.
- Hold for five seconds before releasing.
- Hook your fingers into the corners of your mouth and pull them apart as

wide as you can. Using the muscles
of your mouth, draw your fingers
closer together.

• Do 10 repetitions before releasing.

• Place an index finger at the top of the
nasolabial line, right at the corners of
the nostrils.

• Holding firm, sniff your nose
upwards. Work against the resistance
to strengthen the zygomaticus
muscle.

• Hold for five seconds before
releasing.

• To perform this facial exercise,
please watch the video tutorial at:
**http://bit.ly/nasolabial1 + http://
bit.ly/nasolabial2**

Key acupressure points

The first point to focus on is the Di Cang point. This pressure point is located at the outer edges of the lips, directly below the pupil.

This point is used in cosmetic acupuncture in the treatment of Bell's Palsy in order to lift the face.
- Apply firm pressure with your index or middle fingers
- and make ten small circles before releasing.

The second pressure point is Ying Xiang. While it's primary role is not to reduce nasolabial lines, it will help clear up any sinus or congestion issues around this area.

- This point is located in the nasolabial fold at the corner of the nostril.
- Apply firm pressure and make ten small circles before releasing.

Massage techniques

- Holding your lips over your teeth, form an O with your mouth.
- Run the tips of your index fingers up and down the nasolabial lines.
- With the pads of your index fingers, lightly tap up and down along the nasolabial fold and around the cheeks to increase circulation to the area.
- Rub your hands together to create heat. Place both palms on your cheeks.

- Gently draw your cheeks upwards
  and outwards, smoothing out the
  nasolabial folds.

Chapter 7: Laugh Lines & Lip Fillers

While laugh lines are often confused with the nasolabial folds, this chapter will address the fine lines and wrinkles that form around our lips as we age.

Repeated actions such as drinking through a straw or smoking cigarettes cause the obicularis oris muscles surrounding the lips to fall into these vertical wrinkles.

Fat loss and decreases in collagen production result in less plump lips and thinner, more fragile skin, which combine to make lines more obvious.

True "laugh lines" are the small lines
that form at the sides of the mouth when
we smile.

Vertical lines can also form around the
mouth, colloquially referred to as
"lipstick lines" or "smoker lines". We will
also discuss "marionette lines", the lines
that form from the mouth to the chin.

Facial exercises for laugh lines and lipstick lines

- Place an index finger at each corner of the mouth. Pout your lips and blow kisses to firm the muscles.
- Do ten repetitions before releasing.
- Open your mouth so that your lips are about an inch apart. Slowly bring your upper lip downwards without moving your teeth.

- Hold for five seconds before releasing.
- Place two fingers on your upper lip. Use the muscles of the upper lips to lift the fingers up.
- Hold for five seconds before releasing.
- To perform this facial exercise, please watch the video tutorial at: **http://bit.ly/laughlip**

Strengthen the muscles of your mouth by practicing half smiles.
- Looking in a mirror, keep the right side of your mouth relaxed while smiling with the left side.
- Hold for five seconds before switching sides.

- Tilt your head back, bringing your bottom lip over your teeth. Hold for five seconds before releasing.
- Tilt your head back and make a chewing motion with your jaws.
- Repeat for ten seconds before releasing.
- To perform this facial exercise, please watch the video tutorial at: **http://bit.ly/marionettelines**

Key acupressure points

The Shui Gou point is located at the Cupid's Bow, between the nose and the upper lip. Stimulating this point will reduce fine wrinkles and tone the delicate skin around the lips.

Apply firm pressure with your index
finger and make ten small circles before
releasing.

Massage techniques

The skin around your lips is quite
sensitive so take care to be gentle.
Using a pH Balanced moisturizer or light
oil like Rosehip seed oil will allow your
hands to glide more easily over your
face and mouth, but these maneuvers
can be carried out on dry skin.

Avoid getting any substances on the
mucus membranes of your mouth. Do
not ingest any substances.

- Using the tips of your fingers,
  massage the skin around your lips
  using light circular motions.

- Starting at the middle of your bottom
  lip, move upwards and outwards to
  the edge of your mouth and along the
  top lip.
- Use your index and middle fingers to
  move in firm, upward strokes from
  the edges of your lips out to your
  cheekbones.
- Covering your bottom teeth with your
  lip, rub upwards along the marionette
  lines with the pads of your fingers.
- Increase circulation to the lips by
  applying firm pressure. Using your
  index finger, press into the middle of
  your bottom lip before releasing.
- Work your way around the bottom
  and top lips.

Chapter 8: Define Jaw & Double Chin

Some of the first signs of aging can be seen in the jawline and neck. As we get older, facial skin becomes looser, muscles weaken, and there is a loss of subcutaneous fat, which results in a less defined jawline.

The muscles associated with the jaw are the same muscles that facilitate chewing, namely the masseter, the temporalis, and the medial and lateral pterygoids.

Because these muscles act like scaffolding, we must strengthen these muscles so that they can continue to uphold the face.

A double chin is caused by an accumulation of fat underneath the jaw (although genetics and overall body weight also have an important role to play).

This is accented by the effects of gravity, loose and fragile skin, and a weakened platysma muscle.

The following exercises will work the muscles of the chin and jaw to reshape and redefine a sagging jawline and double chin.

Facial exercise for jaw definition

- Lean your head back and stretch your jaw.
- Make an O shape with your mouth, pretending to your yawn then make chewing motions.
- Repeat each movement for five seconds before releasing.
- Place your hands on either side of your face.
- Move your jaw from left to right, working against the resistance of your hands.
- Do five repetitions on each side before releasing.
- Place three fingers on your chin. Open and close your mouth, working against the resistance of your fingers.
- Do ten repetitions before releasing.

- To perform this facial exercise,
  please watch the video tutorial at:
  http://bit.ly/jawdefinition

Facial exercises for double chin

- Slightly lift your chin up in this holding
  position
- Gently lift your chin up to the ceiling
- Jut your chin up and down with your
  mouth close
- You will be able to see the
  contraction of your vocal muscles on
  your neck
- Repeat for ten repetitions
- Then holding the same position, jut
  your chin up and down but with your
  mouth opening and closing
- Repeat for ten repetitions

- To perform this facial exercise, please watch the video tutorial at: **http://bit.ly/doublechinjut**

Key acupressure points

The Tian Rong point is located in the depression just below the angle of the jaw. Stimulation of this point increases circulation to both the facial nerves and the brain.

- Apply firm pressure with the thumb or middle finger.
- Make ten small circles before releasing.

The second pressure point is the Cheng Jiang point. It is located in the center of the groove just below the lip. Triggering this point invigorates the muscles in the face, mouth, and tongue.

- Apply firm pressure to the area and
  make ten small circles before
  releasing.

Massage techniques

Using a pH Balanced moisturizer or light
oil like Rosehip seed oil will allow your
hands to glide more easily over your
chin and jaw, but this maneuvers can be
carried out on dry skin.

- Using your index fingers, massage in
  circular motions along the jawbone,
  working your way up from the chin to
  the earlobes.
- With your index and middle fingers,
  pinch lightly along the jaw in the
  same direction.
- Repeat the process, gently kneading
  along the jaw with the knuckles of our
  index and middle fingers. Be firm in

your movements but do not go to the
point of pain.

- Using the backs of the hands, make
long, firm strokes from under the chin
to the edge of the jaw.
- Using the backs of the fingers, lightly
tap under the chin and jaw to reduce
a double chin.
- Place your thumbs on your chin and
your fingers behind your ears.
- Use your index fingers to massage
small circles in the depression behind
your earlobes to encourage lymph
drainage from the jaw and chin area.
- Keeping your fingers at your ear,
draw your thumbs firmly up the
jawline, drawing the skin upwards
towards your hands.

Chapter 9: Tighten Neck Skin

There are two dreaded signs of aging that appear on the neck: crepiness and wrinkling, and loose, sagging skin (also known as a "turkey neck".)

The neck is also one of the most difficult places to reduce these telltale signs, but it is possible to revitalize these areas.

The wrinkling, thinning, and sagging of skin is primarily due to a decrease in collagen and elastin. Rapid weight loss can also contribute to loose skin.

As the platysma muscle has a free hanging edge, it is particularly liable to losing tautness as we age. One secret to reducing neck wrinkles is to maintain good posture.

As you go through your day, remember to sit or stand with back straight, chin parallel to the ground, and shoulders back to reduce the lines that appear on the neck from frequently leaning your head down.

Add in the following facial exercises and it won't be long until your skin is firm and beautiful once again.

Exercises for crepey, wrinkling neck skin

- Place your fingers on your neck
- Then jutting your chin forward slightly

- Form a wide smile, hold for five
  seconds before releasing.
- Then lift your chin up towards the
  ceiling and pucker up your lips
- Give the ceiling a big wet kiss and
  stretch out your lips
- Repeat for ten repetitions
- Turn your head to left shoulder, place
  the tip of the tongue on the roof of
  your mouth, smile and swallow.
- Repeat on your right shoulder, place
  the tip of the tongue to the roof of
  your mouth, smile and swallow.
- To perform this facial exercise,
  please watch the video tutorial at:
  http://bit.ly/crepeyneck

Exercises for turkey neck

- Brush your fingers from your neck to
  your chin giving it a slight massage

- Then bring your lower jaw forward and point your chin upwards.
- Place your fingers on your collarbone and bring the corners of your mouth downwards.
- Hold for five seconds before releasing.
- Repeat for ten repetitions
- Watch this video to perform this exercise.
- To perform this facial exercise, please watch the video tutorial at: **http://bit.ly/turtleneck1**

Key acupressure points

The Feng Chi point is located at the base of the skull. Just below the notch of the skull, there is a slight depression with a thin muscle to either side of it.

Place a thumb on each of these muscles and make ten small, firm circles before releasing.

Stimulating this point reduces neck and shoulder tension and keeps you alert, all of which helps you maintain good posture.

Jian Jing is a point located on the top of the shoulder, directly in line with the nipple.

- Use a thumb or knuckle to trigger this point, which gives similar benefits to the Feng Chi point.
- Make ten small circles before releasing.

Massage techniques

Using a pH Balanced moisturizer or light oil like Rosehip seed oil will allow your hands to glide more easily over your neck.

It is particularly advised to moisturize the neck as it does not have as many sebaceous glands as the face, but these maneuvers can be carried out on dry skin if you prefer.

The neck and décolletage are particularly fragile so take care not to damage the skin.

- Using the pads of your fingertips, lean your head back and gently stroke upwards and outwards from the collarbones up to the jaw.

- Repeat this movement on the sides of the neck, starting at the shoulders and working up to the ears.
- Make circular motions with your fingertips across the collarbones and work your way around the décolletage.
- Using both hands, squeeze and knead the shoulders to release tension and pain in the neck and shoulders.

Chapter 10: Step-by-step 8 Minute Routine

This final chapter is a summary of everything you have learnt so far to reduce wrinkles and look 10 years younger.

It recaps what a good facial exercise routine looks like in 8 minutes. This eight minute routine is not exhaustive and not every exercise or tip from the book is included here.

However it is a **comprehensive workout for the face.**

In fact, I suggest you go through the exercises outlined in this book and choose the facial exercises that are relevant to your facial needs.

There are some things that we can't change. We can't turn back time. We can't flip a switch that triggers a cascade of collagen and elastin synthesis.

We can't stop the process of aging. We can, however, aim to reduce the effects of the inevitable.

Younger looking skin is a result of:
- A clean healthy diet that is smoke free
- Strengthening the muscles
- moisturizing the skin
- promoting circulation

- reducing fluid retention
- and training the face not to fall into
  the bad habits that result in persistent
  wrinkles.

8 Minute Routine Break Down By Minute

You can use a pH Balanced moisturizer, light oil like Rosehip seed oil or without oil if you like. However a moisturizer or oil will help your fingers slide more easily over your skin.

** Watch the facial exercise videos again in each chapter to jog your memory before doing this routine.

0:00-0:30

- Place an index finger along each eyebrow.

- Widen your eyes as much as you can
  without your forehead wrinkling. Hold
  for ten seconds before releasing.
- Using light pressure, push your
  brows downwards with your fingers,
  while at the same time, raising your
  eyebrows up.
- Keep your forehead smooth.
- Hold for ten seconds before
  releasing.
- **Combats: worry lines http://bit.ly/
  worrylines**

0:30-1:00

- Place your index and middle fingers
  at the inside of each eyebrow.
- Smooth out any creases in your
  forehead. Hold for ten seconds.
- Use your fingers to hold the skin
  smooth as you attempt to frown.

- Do ten frowning repetitions before releasing.
- **Combats: Frown lines http://bit.ly/frownline**

1:00-1:30

- Place your index fingers at the outer edges of the eye.
- Squeeze the eyes shut and slowly move your fingers out towards your ears. Hold for ten seconds.
- Lightly pull your fingers up as you press your eyelids shut. Hold for ten seconds before releasing.
- Combats: Crow's feet, under eye wrinkles **http://bit.ly/crowfeet**

1:30-2:00

- Squeeze yours eyes tight for three seconds, then open them as wide as possible for three seconds.
- Alternate for thirty seconds before releasing.
- **Combats: Under eye wrinkles, worry lines, frown lines http://bit.ly/undereyewrinkles**

2:00-2:30
- Facing straight ahead, open your mouth in a wide 'O' shape.
- Eyes looking up
- Hold for five seconds before releasing
- Repeat three times
- **Combats: Under eye puffiness and bags http://bit.ly/puffeyebags**

2:30-3:00

- Hook your fingers into the corners of
  your mouth and pull them apart as
  wide as you can.
- Using the muscles of your mouth,
  draw your fingers closer together.
- Do fifteen repetitions before
  releasing.
- **Combats: Sagging cheeks,
  nasolabial folds http://bit.ly/
  nasolabial1 + http://bit.ly/
  nasolabial2**

3:00-3:30

- Tilt your head back, bringing your
  bottom lip over your teeth. Hold for
  ten seconds.
- Keeping your head back, make large
  chewing motions with your jaws.
- Repeat for ten seconds before
  releasing.

- **Combats: Marionette lines, crepiness, sagging jawline http://bit.ly/marionettelines**

3:30-4:00

- Place an index finger at each corner of the mouth.
- Pout your lips and blow kisses.
- Do ten repetitions.
- Looking straight ahead, move your lips up, like you are trying to kiss the ceiling.
- Hold for ten seconds before releasing.
- **Combats: Nasolabial folds, laugh lines, smoker lines**

4:00-4:30

- Puff your cheeks out as far as you can.

- Move the air from the right cheek to the left cheek to the top lip to the bottom lip.
- Hold each position for 4 seconds.
- Complete the cycle twice before releasing.
- **Combats: Nasolabial folds, hollowing cheeks http://bit.ly/hollowcheeks**

4:30-5:00

- Face forward an open your mouth as wide as possible.
- Stick out your tongue and look upwards. Hold for twenty seconds before releasing.
- Combats: Sagging cheeks, under eye puffiness and bags, turkey neck

5:00-5:30

- Place your hands on either side of your face.
- Move your jaw from left to right, working against the resistance of your hands.
- Do ten repetitions on each side before releasing.
- **Combats: Sagging jawline http://bit.ly/jawdefinition**

5:30-6:00

- Jut your chin up and down and you will be able to see the contraction of your vocal muscles
- Do ten repetitions
- **Combats: Double chin http://bit.ly/doublechinjut**

6:00-6:30

- With the tip of your tongue against your mouth, lean your head back. Swallow and smile.
- Repeat the exercise, leaning your head to the right, and then again to the left. Hold each position for ten seconds.
- **Combats: Sagging cheeks, sagging jawline, turkey neck http://bit.ly/crepeyneck**

6:30-7:00

- Place your hands on your forehead.
- Push your head into your hands without letting it move forward.
- Use the resistance to engage the muscles in the neck. Hold for twenty seconds before releasing.
- **Combats: Crepiness, turkey neck http://bit.ly/turtleneck1**

7:00-8:00 (light massage to finish)

- Using moisturizer, oil, or dry hands, make light circular motions with the tips of your fingers.
- Starting at the chin, move upwards and outwards up the jawline, over the cheeks, and across the forehead.
- Move from the bridge of your nose out to the hairline.
- Use lighter pressure to make small circles around the eyes and the lips.
- Using the index, middle and ring fingers at the point of your frown lines, apply light pressure and pull your fingers out towards your temples.
- Repeat this motion from the nostrils across the cheeks, and from the edges of the lips across to the jaw.

- Use long strokes to rub from your collarbone to your jawline. Use the back of your hand to tap firmly under the chin.
- Finally, use the pads of your fingers to lightly tap each area of the face, tapping more gently around the eyes and the lips.
- Finish with light circular strokes, moving from the chin up to the forehead.

That's a wrap! I hope you enjoy 10 Years Younger by using facial exercises.

Remember you **DON'T** have to do facial exercises every day.

Give your face a break as daily facial exercise can be stressful on the skin -

all it takes is 2 - 3 times a week to keep wrinkles at bay.

Take care
Aimee xx

Other Books By Aimee

HEALTH & BEAUTY SERIES

Book 1:
ACNE TREATMENT BOOK - The Adult Acne Treatment Book With Proven Acne Remedies & Treatments To Cure Cystic & Hormonal Acne For Radiant Skin

Book 2:
VOGUE HACKS - The 3 Step Intermittent Fasting System To Lose Up To 10 Pounds In 10 Days & Achieve Rapid Fat Loss.

Book 3:
10 YEARS YOUNGER - Look Younger With Yoga Face Exercises, Get Rid of

Wrinkles & Take 10 Years off Your Face in 8 Mins A Day.

Book 4:

CELLULITE BLASTER - Quick Start Guide To Getting Rid Of Cellulite FAST and Blasting Them Off Your Stomach, Thighs, Legs & Butt!

Simply do a search for "Aimee Blake" on the Amazon Kindle store or visit my Author page at:

http://amazon.com/author/aimeeblake

Free Gift

**Get the "8 Point Facial Acupressure Routine" for Free at:
http://bit.ly/8ptacupressure**

• The facial acupressure routine are for the days you don't want to perform facial exercises.
• The best part it only takes 2 minutes to complete!

**Download it for free now at:
http://bit.ly/8ptacupressure**

About The Author

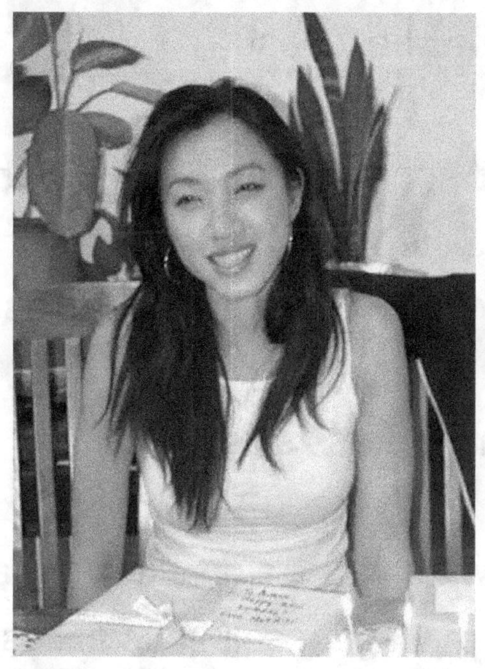

Aimee Blake is from Sydney Australia - she's a self experimenter of all things health, beauty and wellness and is a certified nutritionist.

In October 2013, she lost over 25 pounds in less than 2.5 months without restrictive diets, cardio whilst still eating the foods she loves!

This led her to writing "Vogue Hack" - a simple 3 step weight loss system that helps women with intermittent fasting, losing 10 pounds in 10 days and dropping a dress size fast!

She's written books on skin care and natural anti aging solutions and is committed to helping women all over the world improve their mind, body and spirit.

Thank You... And One Tiny Favor, Please

Thank you for reading my book! I really value your feedback and would appreciate it if you could leave a review.

As an independent author, I have a heart for helping people by sharing the information presented in this book.

Please leave me a helpful review on Amazon right now by going to your kindle store purchases.

It would really help benefit other people and Zeus my doggy values your opinion as well!

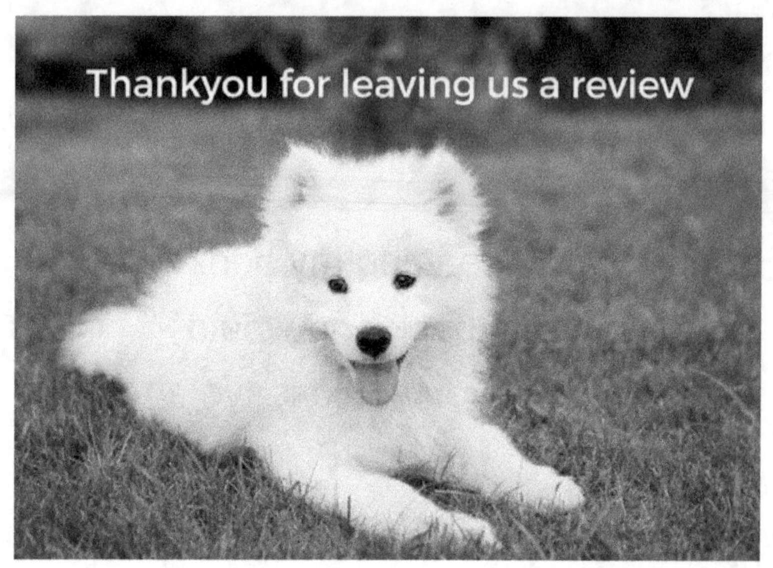
Thankyou for leaving us a review